Air Fryer Seafood Recipes

A Set of Delicious Air Fried Seafood Recipes + Extra Treats

Grace Ward

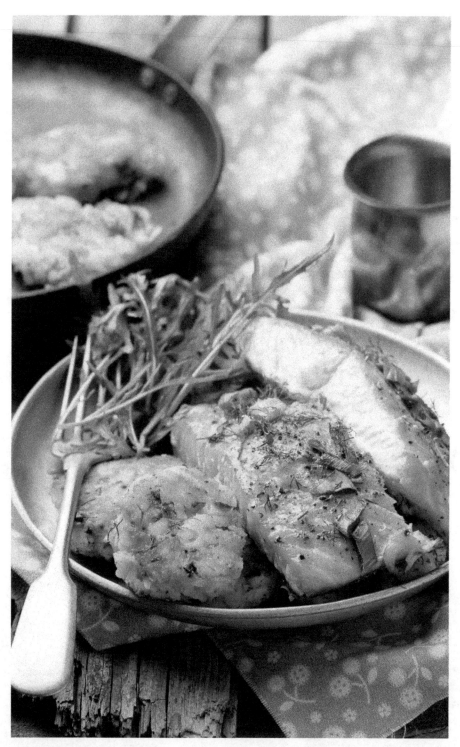

Table of Contents

6

Honey Ginger Salmon Steaks

Cooking time: 10 minutes **Servings**: 2

- 2 salmon steaks
- 2 tablespoons fresh ginger, minced
- 2 garlic cloves, minced
- ¼ cup honey
- 1/3 cup orange juice
- 1/3 cup soy sauce
- 1 lemon, sliced

Directions:

Mix all the Ingredients in a bowl. Marinate the salmon in the sauce for 2-hours in the fridge. Add the marinated salmon to air fryer at 395°fahrenheit for 10-minutes. Garnish with fresh ginger and lemon slices.

NUTRITION: Calories: 514, total Fat: 22g, Carbs : 39.5g, Protein: 41g

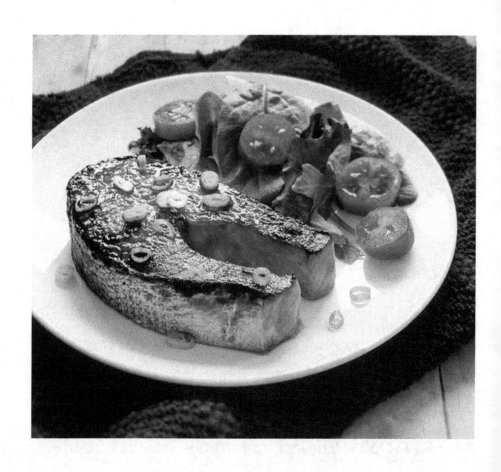

Rosemary & Lemon Salmon

Cooking time: 10 minutes **Servings:** 2

- 2 salmon fillets
- Dash of pepper
- Fresh rosemary, chopped
- 2 slices of lemon

Directions:

Rub the rosemary over your salmon fillets, then season them with salt and pepper, and place lemon slices on top of fillets. Place in the fridge for 2-hours. Preheat your air fryer to 320°fahrenheit. Cook for 10-minutes.

NUTRITION: Calories: 363, total Fat: 22g, Carbs : 8g, Protein: 40g

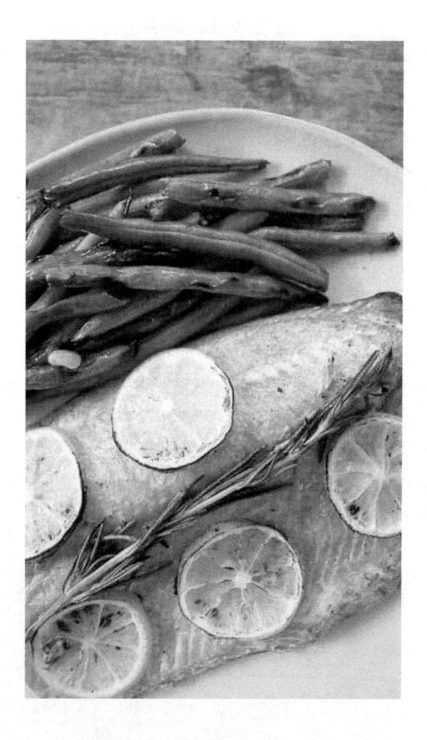

Fish With Capers & Herb Sauce

Cooking time: 15 minutes **Servings:** 4

- 2 cod fillets
- ¼ cup almond flour
- 1 teaspoon dijon mustard
- 1 egg

Sauce:

- 2 tablespoons of light sour cream
- 2 teaspoons capers
- 1 tablespoon tarragon, chopped
- 1 tablespoon fresh dill, chopped
- 2 tablespoons red onion, chopped
- 2 tablespoons dill pickle, chopped

Directions:

Pour in all of the sauce. In a small bowl, add all of the ingredients and stir until well mixed, then chill. In a bowl mix dijon mustard and egg and sprinkle the flour over a plate. Dip the cod fillets first into the egg and coat, then dip them into the flour, coating them on both sides. Preheat your air fryer to 300°fahrenheit, place fillets into air fryer and cook for 10-minutes. Place fillets on serving dishes and drizzle with sauce and serve.

NUTRITION: Calories: 198, total Fat: 9.4g, Carbs : 17.6g, Protein: 11g

Lemon Halibut

Cooking time: 20 minutes **Servings**: 4

- 4 halibut fillets
- 1 egg, beaten
- 1 lemon, sliced
- Salt and pepper to taste
- 1 tablespoon parsley, chopped

Directions:

Sprinkle the lemon juice over the halibut fillets. In a food processor mix the lemon slices, salt, pepper, and parsley. Take fillets and coat them with this mixture; then dip fillets into beaten egg. Cook fillets in your air fryer at 350°fahrenheit for 15-minutes.

NUTRITION: Calories: 48, total Fat: 1g, Carbs : 2.5g, Protein: 9g

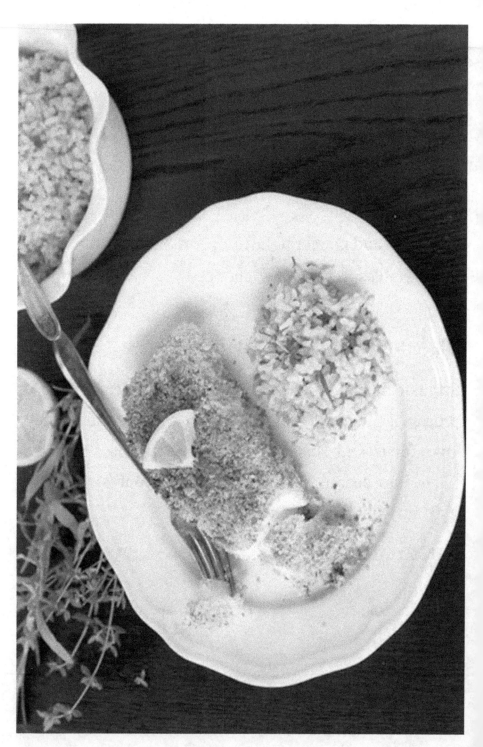

Fried Cod & Spring Onion

Preparation time: 0 minutes **Cooking time**: 20 minutes **Servings**: 4

- 7-ounce cod fillet, washed and dried
- Spring onion, white and green parts, chopped
- A dash of sesame oil
- 5 tablespoons light soy sauce
- 1 teaspoon dark soy sauce
- 3 tablespoons olive oil
- 5 slices of ginger
- 1 cup of water
- Salt and pepper to taste

Directions:

Season the cod fillet with a dash of sesame oil, salt, and pepper. Preheat your air fryer to 356°fahrenheit. Cook the cod fillet in air fryer for 12-minutes. For the seasoning sauce, boil water in a pan on the stovetop, along with both light and dark soy sauce and stir. In another small saucepan, heat the oil and add the ginger and white part of the spring onion. Fry until the ginger browns, then remove the ginger and onions. Top the cod fillet with shredded green onion. Pour the oil over the fillet and add the seasoning sauce on top.

NUTRITION: Calories: 233, total Fat: 16g, Carbs : 15.5g, Protein: 6.7g

Butterflied Prawns With Garlic-Sriracha

Preparation time: 0 minutes **Cooking time**: 15 minutes **Servings:** 2

- 1 tablespoon lime juice
- 1 tablespoon sriracha
- 1-pound large prawns, shells removed and cut lengthwise or
- butterflied
- 1 teaspoon fish sauce
- 2 tablespoons melted butter
- 2 tablespoons minced garlic
- Salt and pepper to taste

Directions:

Preheat the air fryer to 3900 degrees Fahrenheit.

In the air fryer, place the grill pan accessory. Combine the remaining ingredients and season the prawns. Place the pan on the grill and cook for 15 minutes. Ensure that the prawns are turned halfway through the cooking time.

NUTRITION: 443; Carbs :9.7 g; Protein: 62.8g; Fat: 16.9g

Cajun Seasoned Salmon Filet

Cooking time: 15 minutes **Servings:** 1

- 1 salmon fillet
- 1 teaspoon juice from lemon, freshly squeezed
- 3 tablespoons extra virgin olive oil
- A dash of cajun seasoning mix
- Salt and pepper to taste

Directions:

Preheat the air fryer for 5 minutes. In a mixing bowl, combine all of the ingredients and cover. In the air fryer basket, position the fish fillet. Bake for 15 minutes at 3250f. Once cooked drizzle with olive oil

NUTRITION: 523; Carbohydrates: 4.6g; Protein: 47.9g; Fat: 34.8g

Cajun Spiced Veggie-Shrimp Bake

Preparation time: 0 minutes **Cooking time**: 20 minutes **Servings**: 4

- 1 bag of frozen mixed vegetables
- 1 tbsp gluten free cajun seasoning
- Olive oil spray
- Season with salt and pepper
- Small shrimp peeled & deveined (regular size bag about 50-80 small shrimp)

Directions:

Cooking spray the baking pan of the air fryer lightly. Toss all of the ingredients together to coat. Season generously with pepper and salt. For 10 minutes, cook on 330of. Halfway through Cooking time, stir. Cook for 10 minutes at 330of.

NUTRITION: 78; Carbs : 13.2g; Protein: 2.8g; Fat: 1.5g

Air Fried Cod With Basil Vinaigrette

Servings:*4*

- ¼ cup olive oil
- 3cod fillets
- A bunch of basil, torn
- Juice from 1 lemon, freshly squeezed
- Salt and pepper *to taste*

Directions:

1.Preheat the air fryer for 5 minutes.

2.Season the cod fillets with salt and pepper to taste.

3.Place in the air fryer and cook for 15 minutes at 3500f.

4.Meanwhile, mix the rest of the in a bowl and toss to combine.

5.Serve the air fried cod with the basil vinaigrette.

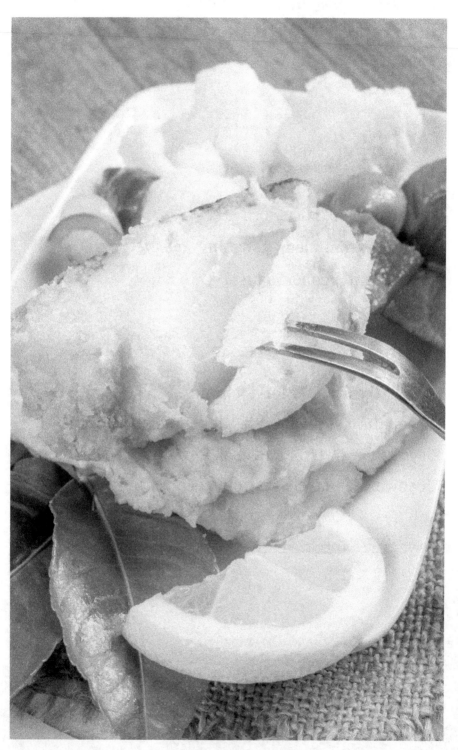

Almond Flour Coated Crispy Shrimps

Servings: 4

- ½ cup almond flour
- 1tablespoon yellow mustard
- 1-pound raw shrimps, peeled and deveined
- 3 tablespoons olive oil
- Salt and pepper to taste

Directions:

1.Place all in a ziploc bag and give a good shake.

2.Place in the air fryer and cook for 10 minutes at 4000f.

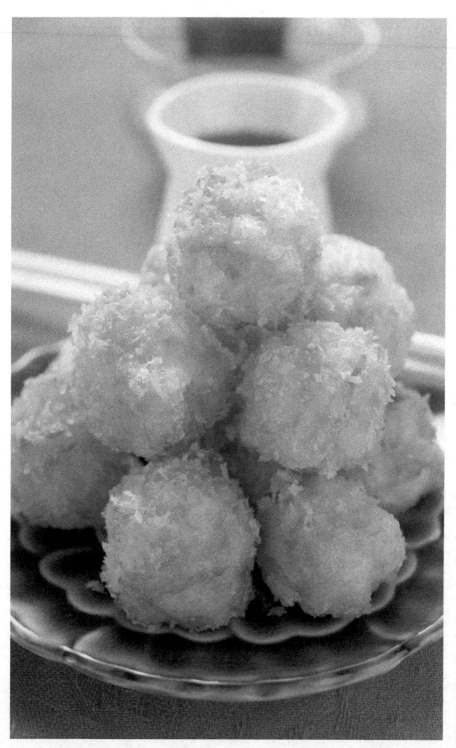

Apple Slaw Topped Alaskan Cod Filet

Servings: 3

- ¼ cup mayonnaise
- ½ red onion, diced
- 1½ pounds frozen alaskan cod
- 1box whole wheat panko breadcrumbs
- 1 granny smith apple, julienned
- 1tablespoon vegetable oil
- 1 teaspoon paprika
- 2cups napa cabbage, shredded
- Salt and pepper to taste

Directions:

1.Preheat the air fryer to 390of.

2.Place the grill pan accessory in the air fryer.

3.Brush the fish with oil and dredge in the breadcrumbs.

4.Place the fish on the grill pan and cook for 15 minutes. Make sure to flip the fish halfway through the Cooking time.

5.Meanwhile, prepare the slaw by mixing the remaining in a bowl.

6.Serve the fish with the slaw.

Baked Cod Fillet Recipe From Thailand

Servings: 4

- ¼ cup coconut milk, freshly squeezed
- 1 tablespoon lime juice, freshly squeezed
- 1-pound cod fillet, cut into bite-sized pieces
- Salt and pepper to taste

Directions:

1.Preheat the air fryer for 5 minutes.

2.Place all in a baking dish that will fit in the air fryer.

3.Place in the air fryer.

4.Cook for 20 minutes at 3250f.

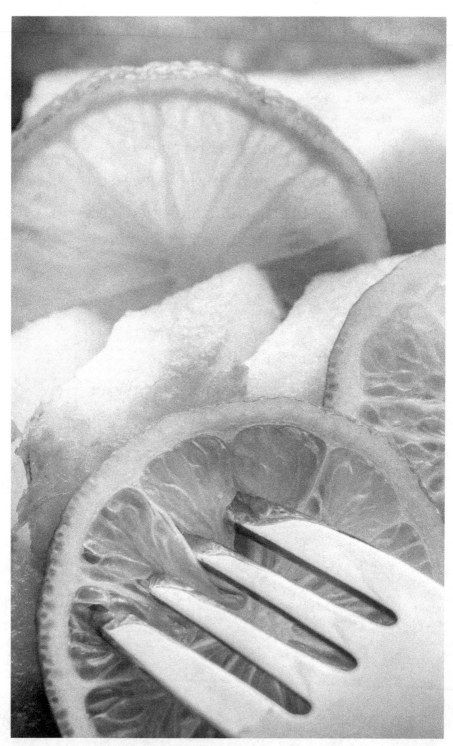

Baked Scallops With Garlic Aioli

Servings: 4

- 1 cup breadcrumbs
- 1/4 cup chopped parsley
- 16 sea scallops, rinsed and drained
- 2 shallots, chopped
- 3 pinches ground nutmeg
- 4 tablespoons olive oil
- 5 cloves garlic, minced
- 5 tablespoons butter, melted
- Salt and pepper to taste

Directions:

1.Lightly grease baking pan of air fryer with Cooking spray.

2.Mix in shallots, garlic, melted butter, and sCal lops. Season with pepper, salt, and nutmeg.

3.In a small bowl, whisk well olive oil and breadcrumbs. Sprinkle

4.over sCal lops.

5.For 10 minutes, cook on 390of until tops are lightly browned.

6.Serve and enjoy with a sprinkle of parsley.

Basil 'N Lime-Chili Clams

Servings: 3

- ½ cup basil leaves
- ½ cup tomatoes, chopped
- 1tablespoon fresh lime juice
- 25 littleneck clams
- 4cloves of garlic, minced
- 6tablespoons unsalted butter
- Salt and pepper to taste

Directions:

1. Preheat the air fryer to 390 0f.

    1. Place the grill pan accessory in the air fryer.

    2. On a large foil, place all . Fold over the foil and close by crimping the edges.

    3. Place on the grill pan and cook for 15 minutes.

    4. Serve with bread.

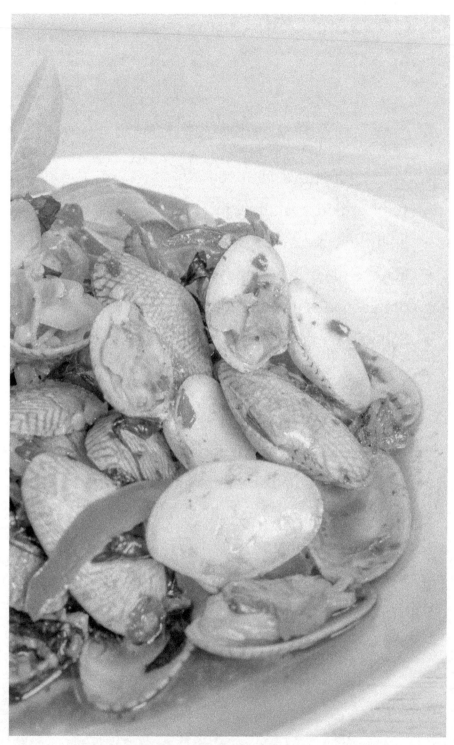

Bass Filet In Coconut Sauce

Servings:4

- ¼ cup coconut milk
- ½ pound bass fillet
- 1 tablespoon olive oil
- 2 tablespoons jalapeno, chopped
- 2 tablespoons lime juice, freshly squeezed
- 3 tablespoons parsley, chopped
- Salt and pepper to taste

Directions:

1.Preheat the air fryer for 5 minutes

2.Season the bass with salt and pepper to taste

3.Brush the surface with olive oil.

4.Place in the air fryer and cook for 15 minutes at 3500f.

5. Meanwhile, place in a saucepan, the coconut milk, lime juice, jalapeno and parsley.

6.Heat over medium flame.

7.Serve the fish with the coconut sauce.

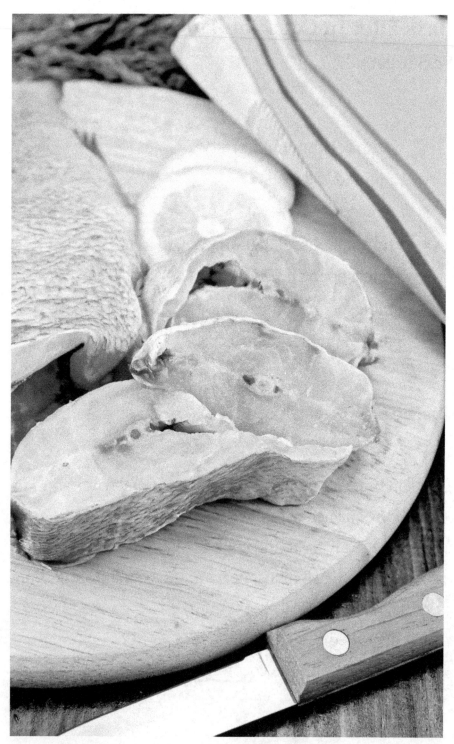

Beer Battered Cod Filet

Servings: 2

- ½ cup all-purpose flour
- ¾ teaspoon baking powder
- 1 ¼ cup lager beer
- 2cod fillets
- 2eggs, beaten
- Salt and pepper to taste

Directions:

1.Preheat the air fryer to 3900f.

2.Pat the fish fillets dry then set aside.

3.In a bowl, combine the rest of the to create a batter.

4.Dip the fillets on the batter and place on the double layer rack.

5.Cook for 15 minutes.

Buttered Baked Cod With Wine

Servings: 2

- 1tablespoon butter
- 1tablespoon butter
- 2tablespoons dry white wine
- 1/2 pound thick-cut cod loin
- 1-1/2 teaspoons chopped fresh parsley
- 1-1/2 teaspoons chopped green onion
- 1/2 lemon, cut into wedges
- 1/4 sleeve buttery round crackers (such as ritz®), crushed
- 1/4 lemon, juiced

Directions:

1.In a small bowl, melt butter in microwave. Whisk in crackers.

2.Lightly grease baking pan of air fryer with remaining butter. And melt for 2 minutes at 390of.

3.In a small bowl whisk well lemon juice, white wine, parsley, and

4.green onion.

5.Coat cod filets in melted butter. Pour dressing. Top with buttercracker mixture.

6.Cook for 10 minutes at 390of.

7.Serve and enjoy with a slice of lemon.

Buttered Garlic-Oregano On Clams

Servings: 4

- ¼ cup parmesan cheese, grated
- ¼ cup parsley, chopped
- 1 cup breadcrumbs
- 1teaspoon dried oregano
- 2 dozen clams, shucked
- 3cloves of garlic, minced
- 4tablespoons butter, melted

Directions:

1.In a medium bowl, mix the breadcrumbs, parmesan cheese, parsley, oregano, and garlic. Stir in the melted butter.

2.Preheat the air fryer to 3900f.

3.Place the baking dish accessory in the air fryer and place the clams.

4.Sprinkle the crumb mixture over the clams.

5. Cook for 5 minutes.

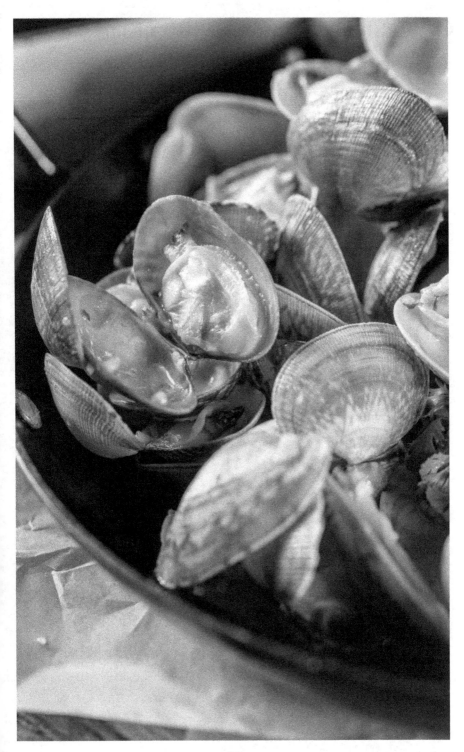

Cajun Spiced Lemon-Shrimp Kebabs

Servings: 2

- 1tsp cayenne
- 1tsp garlic powder
- 1 tsp kosher salt
- 1tsp onion powder
- 1 tsp oregano
- 1tsp paprika
- 12pcs xl shrimp
- 2lemons, sliced thinly crosswise
- 2 tbsp olive oil

Directions:

1.In a bowl, mix all Ingredients except for sliced lemons. Marinate for 10 minutes.

2.Thread 3 shrimps per steel skewer.

3.Place in skewer rack.

4.Cook for 5 minutes at 390of.

5.Serve and enjoy with freshly squeezed lemon.

Panko-Crusted Tilapia

Servings: 3

- 2tsp. Italian seasoning
- 2tsp. Lemon pepper
- 1/3 c. Panko breadcrumbs
- 1/3 c. Egg whites
- 1/3 c. Almond flour
- 3 tilapia fillets Olive oil

Directions:

1. Place panko, egg whites, and flour into separate bowls. Mix lemon pepper and italian seasoning in with breadcrumbs.

1. Pat tilapia fillets dry. Dredge in flour, then egg, breadcrumb mixture.

2. Add to the air fryer basket and spray lightly with olive oil.

3. Cook 10-11 minutes at 400 degrees, making sure to flip halfway through Cooking .

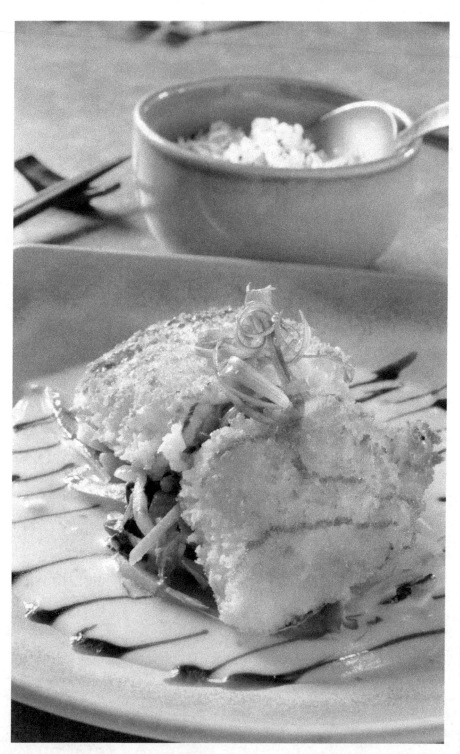

Coconut Shrimp

Servings: 3

- 1c. Almond flour
- 1c. Panko breadcrumbs
- 1 tbsp. Coconut flour
- 1c. Unsweetened, dried coconut
- 1 egg white
- 12 raw large shrimp

Directions:

1.Put shrimp on paper towels to drain.

2.Mix coconut and panko breadcrumbs. Then mix in coconut flour and almond flour in a different bowl. Set to the side.

3.Dip shrimp into flour mixture, then into egg white, and then into coconut mixture.

4.Place into air fryer basket. Repeat with remaining shrimp.

5.Set temperature to 350°f and set time to 10 minutes. Turn halfway through Cooking process.

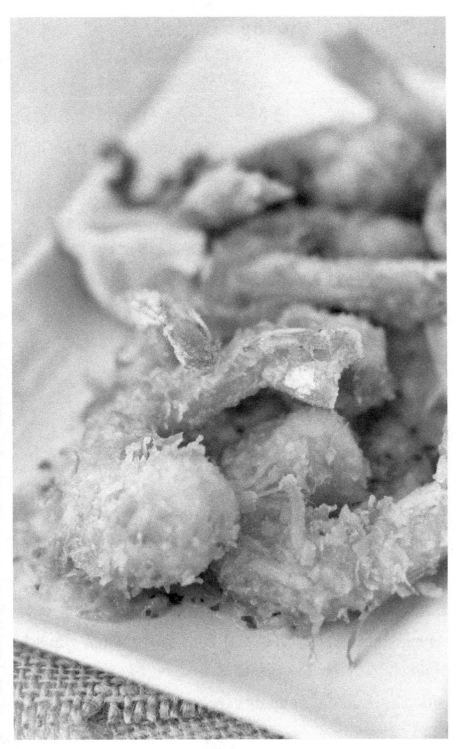

Scallops And Spring Veggies

Servings: 4

- ½ pound asparagus, ends trimmed, cut into 2-inch pieces
- 1 cup Sugar snap peas
- 1-pound sea Scallops
- 1tablespoon lemon juice
- 1 teaspoons olive oil
- ½ teaspoon dried thyme
- Pinch salt
- Freshly ground black pepper

Directions:

1.Place the asparagus and Sugar snap peas in the air fryer basket.

2.Cook for 2 to 3 minutes or until the vegetables are just starting to get tender.

3.Meanwhile, check the sCal lops for a small muscle attached to the

4.side, and pull it off and discard.

5.In a medium bowl, toss the sCal lops with the lemon juice, olive oil, thyme, salt, and pepper. Place into the air fryer oven basket on top of the vegetables.

6.Steam for 5 to 7 minutes, tossing the basket once during cooking time, until the sCal lops are just firm when tested with your finger and are opaque in the center, and the vegetables are tender. Serve immediately.

Air Fryer Salmon Patties

Servings: 4

- 1tbsp. Olive oil
- 1 tbsp. Ghee
- ¼ tsp. Salt
- 1/8 tsp. Pepper
- 1 egg
- 1c. Almond flour
- 1can wild alaskan pink salmon

Directions:

1.Drain can of salmon into a bowl and keeps liquid. Discard skin and bones.

2.Add salt, pepper, and egg to salmon, mixing well with hands to incorporate. Make patties.

3.Dredge in flour and remaining egg. If it seems dry, spoon reserved salmon liquid from the can onto patties.

4.Pour the patties into the oven rack/basket. Place the rack on the

5.middle-shelf of the air fryer oven. Set temperature to

378°f and set time to 7 minutes. Cook 7 minutes till golden, making sure to flip once during cooking process.

Beer-Battered Fish And Chips

Servings: 4

- 2eggs
- 1cup malty beer, such as pabst blue ribbon
- 1 cup all-purpose flour
- ½ cup cornstarch
- 1teaspoon garlic powder
- Salt
- Pepper Cooking oil
- (4-ounce) cod fillets

Directions:

1.In a medium bowl, beat the eggs with the beer. In another medium bowl, combine the flour and cornstarch, and season with the garlic powder and salt and pepper to taste.

2.Spray the air fryer basket with cooking oil.

3.Dip each cod fillet in the flour and cornstarch mixture and then in the egg and beer mixture. Dip the cod in the flour and cornstarch a second time.

4.2 place the cod in the air fryer oven. Do not stack. Cook in batches.

5.Spray with cooking oil. Cook for 8 minutes.

6.Open the air fryer oven and flip the cod. Cook for an additional 7 minutes.

7.Remove the cooked cod from the air fryer, repeat steps 4 and 5 for the remaining fillets.

8.Serve with prepared air fried frozen fries. Frozen fries will need to be

9.cooked for 18 to 20 minutes at 400°f.

10.Cool before serving.

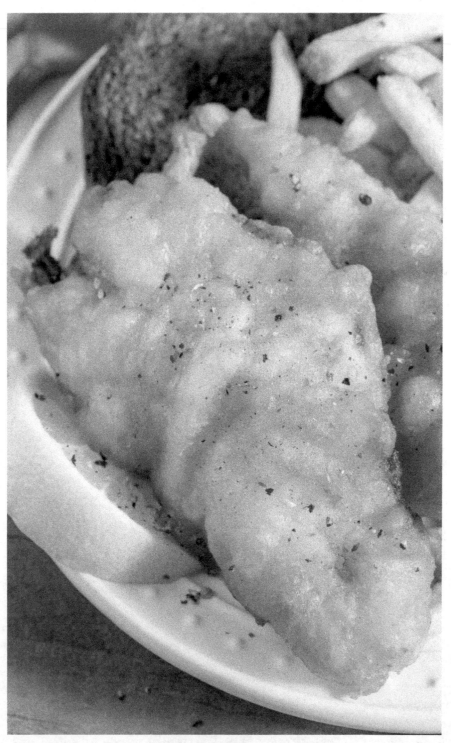

Air Fryer Salmon

Servings: 2

- ½ tsp. Salt
- ½ tsp. Garlic powder
- ½ tsp. Smoked paprika Salmon

Directions:

1. Mix spices and sprinkle onto salmon.

2. Place seasoned salmon into the air fryer oven.

3. Pour into the oven rack/basket. Place the rack on the middle-shelf of the air fryer oven. Set temperature to 400°f and set time to 10 minutes.

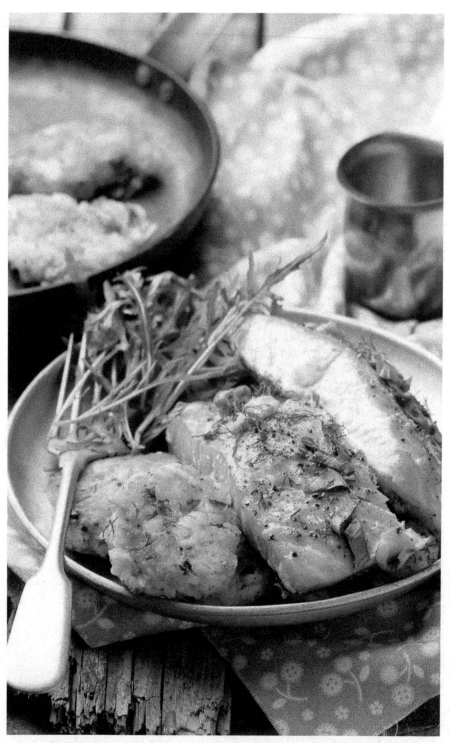

Indian Fish Fingers

Servings: 4

- 1/2-pound fish fillet
- 1tablespoon finely chopped fresh mint leaves or any fresh herbs
- 1/3 cup breadcrumbs
- 1teaspoon ginger garlic paste or ginger and garlic powders
- 1 hot green chili finely chopped
- 1/2 teaspoon paprika
- Generous pinch of black pepper
- Salt to taste
- 3/4 tablespoons lemon juice
- 3/4 teaspoons garam masala powder
- 1/3 teaspoon rosemary
- 1egg

Directions:

1.Start by removing any skin on the fish, washing, and patting dry. Cut the fish into fingers.

2.In a medium bowl mix all except for fish, mint, and breadcrumbs. Bury the fingers in the mixture and refrigerate for 30 minutes.

3.Remove from the bowl from the fridge and mix in mint leaves.

4.In a separate bowl beat the egg, pour breadcrumbs into a third bowl. Dip the fingers in the egg bowl then toss them in the breadcrumbs bowl.

5.Pour into the oven rack/basket. Place the rack on the middle-shelf of the air fryer oven. Set temperature to 360°f, and set time to 15 minutes, toss the fingers halfway through.

Quick Paella

Servings: 4

- 1(10-ounce) package frozen cooked rice, thawed
- (6-ounce) jar artichoke hearts, drained and chopped
- ¼ cup vegetable broth
- ½ teaspoon turmeric
- ½ teaspoon dried thyme
- cup frozen cooked small shrimp
- ½ cup frozen baby peas 1 tomato, diced

Directions:

1.In a 6-by-6-by-2-inch pan, combine the rice, artichoke hearts, vegetable broth, turmeric, and thyme, and stir gently.

2.Place in the air fryer oven and bake for 8 to 9 minutes or until the rice is hot. Remove from the air fryer and gently stir in the shrimp, peas, and tomato. Cook for 5 to 8 minutes or until the shrimp and peas are hot and the paella is bubbling.

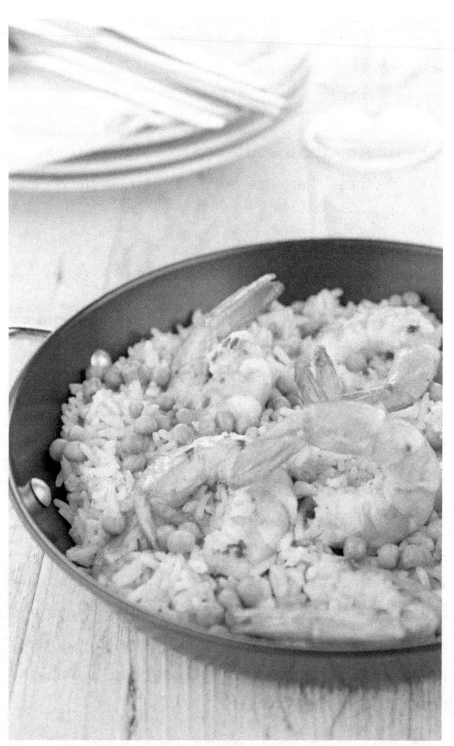

3-Ingredient Air Fryer Catfish

Servings: 4

- 1 tbsp. Chopped parsley
- 1 tbsp. Olive oil
- ¼ c. Seasoned fish fry
- 4 catfish fillets

Directions:

1.Ensure your air fryer oven is preheated to 400 degrees.

2.Rinse off catfish fillets and pat dry.

3.Add fish fry seasoning to ziploc baggie, then catfish. Shake bag and ensure fish gets well coated.

4.Spray each fillet with olive oil.

5.Add fillets to air fryer basket.

6.Set temperature to 400°f and set time to 10 minutes.

7.Cook 10 minutes. Then flip and cook another 2-3 minutes.

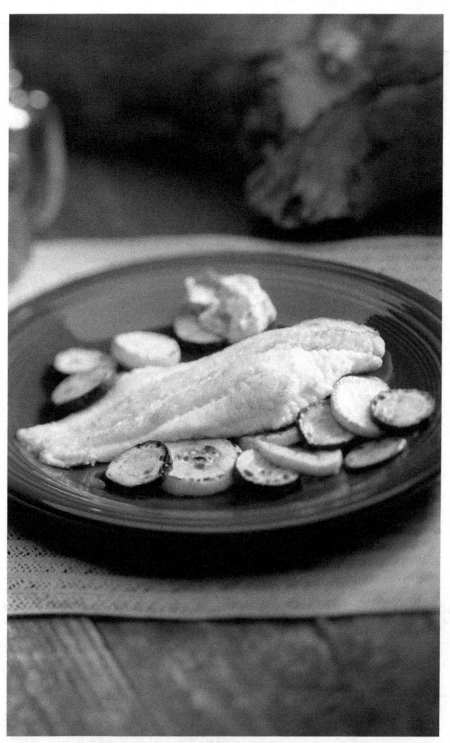

Tuna Veggie Stir-Fry

Servings: 4

- 1tablespoon olive oil
- 1red bell pepper, chopped
- 1cup green beans, cut into 2-inch pieces
- 1 onion, sliced
- 2cloves garlic, sliced
- 2tablespoons low-Sodium soy sauce
- 1 tablespoon honey
- ½ pound fresh tuna, cubed

Directions:

1.In a 6-inch metal bowl, combine the olive oil, pepper, green beans, onion, and garlic.

2.Pour into the oven rack/basket. Place the rack on the middle-shelf of the air fryer oven. Set temperature to 350°f, and set time to 4 to 6 minutes, stirring once, until crisp and tender. Add soy sauce, honey, and tuna, and stir. Cook for another 3 to 6 minutes, stirring once, until the tuna is cooked as desired. Tuna can be served rare or medium-rare, or you can cook it until well done.

Bang Panko Breaded Fried Shrimp

Servings: 4

- 1tsp. Paprika
- Montreal chicken seasoning
- ¾ c. Panko breadcrumbs
- ½ c. Almond flour
- 1 egg white
- 1-pound raw shrimp (peeled and deveined)

Bang bang sauce:

- ¼ c. Sweet chili sauce
- tbsp. Sriracha sauce
- 1/3 c. Plain greek yogurt

Directions:

1. Ensure your air fryer oven is preheated to 400 degrees.

2. Season all shrimp with seasonings.

3. Add flour to one bowl, egg white in another, and breadcrumbs to a third.

4. Dip seasoned shrimp in flour, then egg whites, and then breadcrumbs.

5.Spray coated shrimp with olive oil and add to air fryer basket.

6.Set temperature to 400°f and set time to 4 minutes. Cook 4 minutes, flip, and cook an additional 4 minutes.

7.To make the sauce, mix all sauce until smooth.

Louisiana Shrimp Po Boy

Servings: 6

- 1tsp. Creole seasoning
- 8 slices of tomato
- Lettuce leaves
- ¼ c. Buttermilk
- ½ c. Louisiana fish fry
- 1-pound deveined shrimp remoulade sauce:
- 1chopped green onion
- 1 tsp. Hot sauce
- 1tsp. Dijon mustard
- ½ tsp. Creole seasoning
- 1tsp. Worcestershire sauce
- Juice of ½ a lemon
- ½ c. Vegan mayo

Directions:

1.To make the sauce, combine all sauce until well incorporated. Chill while you cook shrimp.

2.Mix seasonings together and liberally season shrimp.

3.Add buttermilk to a bowl. Dip each shrimp into milk and place in a ziploc bag. Chill half an hour to marinate.

4.Add fish fry to a bowl. Take shrimp from marinating bag and dip into fish fry, then add to air fryer.

5.Ensure your air fryer is preheated to 400 degrees.

6.Spray shrimp with olive oil.

7.Pour into the oven rack/basket. Place the rack on the middle-shelf of the air fryer oven. Set temperature to 400°f and set time to 5 minutes. Cook 5 minutes, flip and then cook another 5 minutes. Assemble "keto" po boy by adding sauce to lettuce leaves, along with shrimp and tomato.

Old Bay Crab Cakes

Servings: 4

- Slices dried bread, crusts removed Small amount of milk
- 1tablespoon mayonnaise
- 1tablespoon worcestershire sauce
- 1 tablespoon baking powder
- 1tablespoon parsley flakes
- 1teaspoon old bay® seasoning
- 1/4 teaspoon salt
- 1egg
- 1-pound lump crabmeat

Directions:

1.Crush your bread over a large bowl until it is broken down into small pieces. Add milk and stir until breadcrumbs are moistened. Mix in mayo and worcestershire sauce. Add remaining and mix well. Shape into 4 patties.

2.Pour into the oven rack/basket. Place the rack on the middle-shelf of the air fryer oven. Set temperature to 360°f, and set time to 20 minutes, flip halfway through.

Flavors Parmesan Shrimp

Servings: 3

- 1lb. Shrimp, peeled and deveined
- 1 tbsp olive oil
- 1/2 tsp onion powder
- 1/2 tsp basil
- 1/4 tsp oregano
- 1/2 tsp pepper
- 1/4 cup parmesan cheese, grated
- 3 garlic cloves, minced

Directions:

1. Add all into the large bowl and toss well.

2. Line instant pot multi-level air fryer basket with aluminum foil.

3. Add shrimp into the air fryer basket and place basket into the instant pot.

4. Seal pot with air fryer lid and select air fry mode then set the temperature to 350 f and timer for 10 minutes.

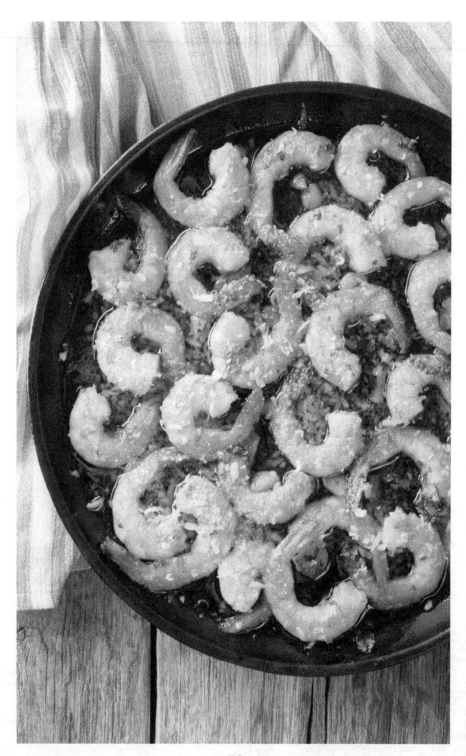

Bacon Wrap Shrimp

Servings: 2

- 8 shrimp, deveined
- 8 bacon slices

Directions:

1.Place the dehydrating tray in a multi-level air fryer basket and place basket in the instant pot.

2.Wrap shrimp with bacon slices and place on dehydrating tray.

3.Seal pot with air fryer lid and select air fry mode then set the temperature to 390 f and timer for 7 minutes. Turn shrimp after 5 minutes.

4.Serve and enjoy.

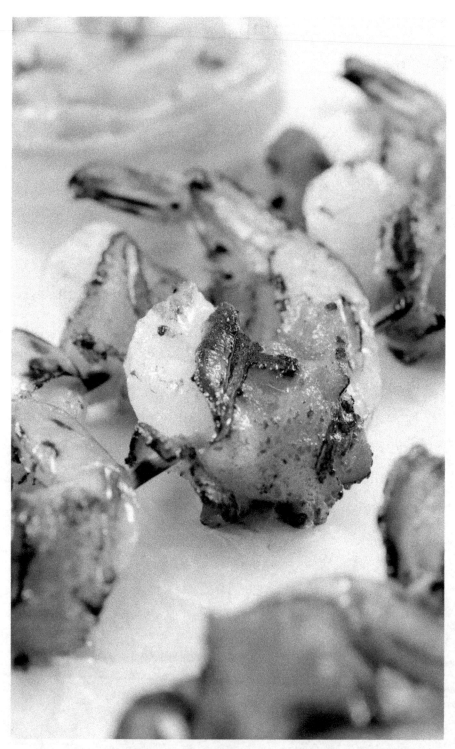

Simple Garlic Lime Shrimp

Servings: 2

- 1cup shrimp
- 1garlic clove, minced
- 1 fresh lime juice
- Pepper
- Salt

Directions:

1.Add all into the bowl and toss well.

2.Spray instant pot multi-level air fryer basket with Cooking spray.

3.Add shrimp into the air fryer basket and place basket into the instant pot.

4.Seal pot with air fryer lid and select air fry mode then set the temperature to 350 f and timer for 8 minutes. Turn shrimp halfway through.

5.Serve and enjoy.

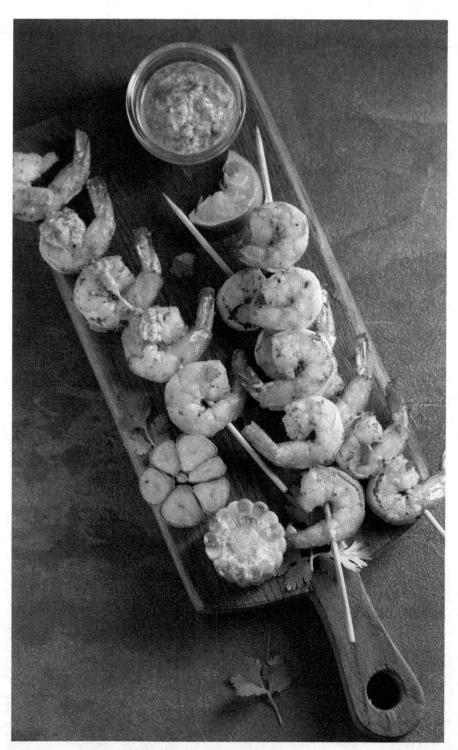

Lemon Crab Patties

Servings: 4

- 1 egg
- 12 oz crabmeat
- 2 green onion, chopped
- 1/4 cup mayonnaise
- cup almond flour
- 1 tsp old bay seasoning
- 1 tsp red pepper flakes
- 1 tbsp fresh lemon juice

Directions:

1. Add half almond flour into the shallow bowl.

2. add remaining and mix until well combined.

3. Place the dehydrating tray in a multi-level air fryer basket and place basket in the instant pot.

4. Make patties and coat with remaining almond flour and place on dehydrating tray.

5.Seal pot with air fryer lid and select air fry mode then set the temperature to 400 f and timer for 10 minutes. Turn patties halfway through.

6.Serve and enjoy.

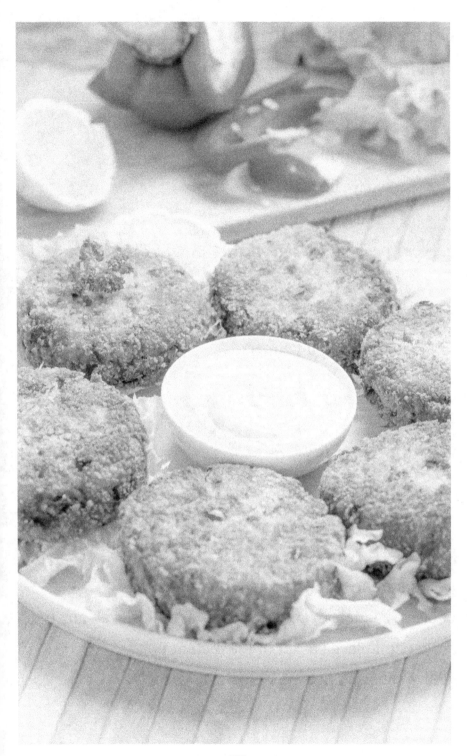

Cheese Crust Salmon

Servings: 2

- 2salmon fillets
- 2tbsp fresh parsley, chopped
- 1 garlic clove, minced
- 1/4 cup parmesan cheese, shredded
- 1/2 tsp mccormick's bbq seasoning
- 1/2 tsp paprika
- 1tbsp olive oil Pepper
- Salt

Directions:

1.Add salmon, seasoning, and olive oil to the bowl and mix well.

2.Mix cheese, garlic, and parsley.

3.Sprinkle cheese mixture on top of salmon.

4.Place the dehydrating tray in a multi-level air fryer basket and place basket in the instant pot.

5.Place salmon fillets on dehydrating tray.

6.Seal pot with air fryer lid and select air fry mode then set the temperature to 400 f and timer for 10 minutes.

7.Serve and enjoy.

Lemon Butter Salmon

Servings: 2

- 2salmon fillets
- 1tsp olive oil
- 2tsp garlic, minced
- 2 tbsp butter
- 2tbsp fresh lemon juice
- 1/4 cup white wine
- Pepper
- Salt

Directions:

1.Place the dehydrating tray in a multi-level air fryer basket and place basket in the instant pot.

2.Season salmon with pepper and salt and place on dehydrating tray.

3.Seal pot with air fryer lid and select air fry mode then set the temperature to 350 f and timer for 6 minutes.

4.Meanwhile, in a saucepan, add remaining and cook over low heat for 5 minutes.

5.Place cooked salmon fillets on serving dish and pour prepared sauce over salmon.

6.Serve and enjoy.

Tasty Spicy Shrimp

Servings: 2

- 1/2 lb. Shrimp, peeled and deveined
- 1/2 tsp old bay seasoning
- 1/4 tsp cayenne pepper
- 1tbsp olive oil
- 1/4 tsp paprika
- 1/8 tsp salt

Directions:

Add all into the mixing bowl and toss well.

Spray instant pot multi-level air fryer basket with Cooking spray.

Add shrimp into the air fryer basket and place basket into the instant pot.

Seal pot with air fryer lid and select air fry mode then set the temperature to 390 f and timer for 6 minutes.

Serve and enjoy.

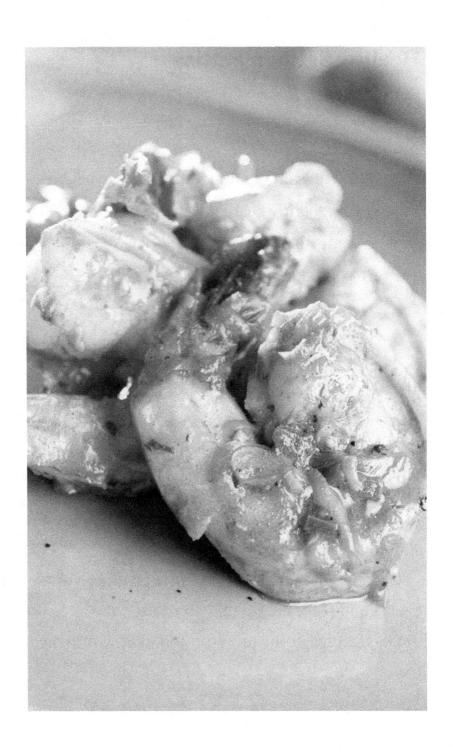

Healthy Salmon Patties

Servings: 4

- 14oz can salmon, drained and remove bones
- 2 eggs, lightly beaten
- 1/2 cup almond flour
- 1/2 onion, minced
- 1/4 cup butter
- 1/2 tsp pepper
- 1 avocado, diced
- 1 tsp salt

Directions:

1.Add all into the mixing bowl and mix until well combined.

2.Place the dehydrating tray in a multi-level air fryer basket and place basket in the instant pot.

3.Make patties from mixture and place on dehydrating tray.

4.Seal pot with air fryer lid and select air fry mode then set the temperature to 400 f and timer for 10 minutes. Turn patties halfway through.

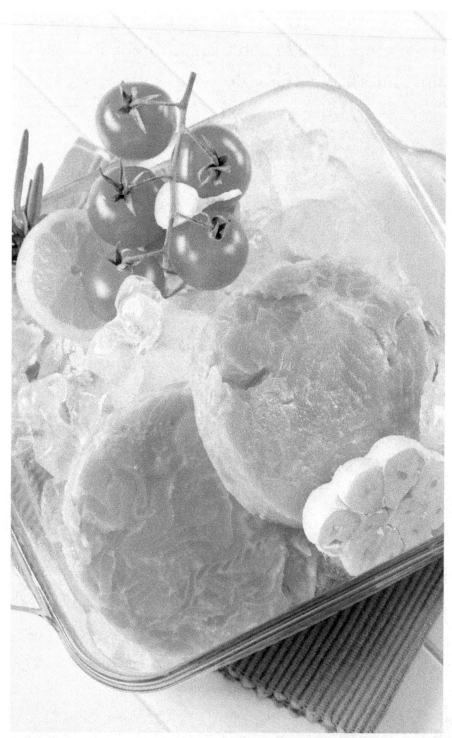

Lemon Garlicky Shrimp

Servings: 4

- 1lb. Shrimp, peeled
- 1 tbsp olive oil
- 1lemon juice
- 1lemon zest
- 1/4 cup fresh parsley, chopped
- 4 garlic cloves, minced
- 1/4 tsp red pepper flakes
- 1/4 tsp sea salt

Directions:

1. Add all   except parsley and lemon juice into the mixing
1. bowl and toss well.
2. Spray instant pot multi-level air fryer basket with Cooking spray.
3. Add shrimp into the air fryer basket and place basket into the instant pot.

4.Seal pot with air fryer lid and select air fry mode then set the

5.temperature to 400 f and timer for 5 minutes.

6.Garnish shrimp with parsley and drizzle with lemon juice.

7.Serve and enjoy.

Spicy Prawns

Servings: 4

- 12 king prawns
- 1/4 tsp black pepper
- 1 tsp chili powder
- 1 tsp red chili flakes
- 1 tbsp vinegar
- 1 tbsp ketchup
- 3 tbsp mayonnaise
- 1/2 tsp sea salt

Directions:

1. Add prawns, chili flakes, chili powder, black pepper, and salt to the bowl and toss well.

2. Spray instant pot multi-level air fryer basket with cooking spray.

3. Add shrimp into the air fryer basket and place basket into the instant pot.

4.Seal pot with air fryer lid and select air fry mode then set the temperature to 350 f and timer for 6 minutes. Stir halfway through.

5.In a small bowl, mix mayonnaise, ketchup, and vinegar.

6.Serve shrimp with mayo mixture.

Simple & Perfect Salmon

Servings: 2

- 2 salmon fillets, remove any bones
- 2 tsp olive oil
- 2tsp paprika
- Pepper
- Salt

Directions:

1. Coat salmon with oil and season with paprika, pepper, and salt.

2. Place the dehydrating tray in a multi-level air fryer basket and place basket in the instant pot.

3. Place salmon fillets on dehydrating tray.

4. Seal pot with air fryer lid and select air fry mode then set the temperature to 390 f and timer for 7 minutes.

5. Serve and enjoy.

Crispy Crust Ranch Fish Fillets

Servings: 2

- 2fish fillets
- 1/2packet ranch dressing mix
- 1/4 cup breadcrumbs
- 1 egg, lightly beaten
- 1 1/4 tbsp olive oil

Directions:

1.In a shallow dish mix together ranch dressing mix and breadcrumbs.

2.Add oil and mix until the mixture becomes crumbly.

3.Place the dehydrating tray in a multi-level air fryer basket and place basket in the instant pot.

4.Dip fish fillet in egg then coats with breadcrumb and place on dehydrating tray.

5.Seal pot with air fryer lid and select air fry mode then set the temperature to 350 f and timer for 12 minutes. Turn fish fillets halfway through.

6.Serve and enjoy.

Sweet Cod Fillets

Servings: 4

- 4 cod fillets, boneless
- Salt and black pepper to taste
- 1 cup water
- 4tablespoons light soy sauce
- 1 tablespoon Sugar
- 3tablespoons olive oil + a drizzle
- 4ginger slices
- 3spring onions, chopped
- 2tablespoons coriander, chopped

Directions:

1.Season the fish with salt and pepper, then drizzle some oil over it and rub well.

2.Put the fish in your air fryer and cook at 360 degrees f for 12 minutes.

3.Put the water in a pot and heat up over medium heat; add the soy sauce and Sugar, stir, bring to a simmer, and remove from the heat.

4.Heat a pan with the olive oil over medium heat; add the ginger and green onions, stir, cook for 2-3 minutes, and remove from the heat.

5.Divide the fish between plates and top with ginger, coriander, and green onions.

6.Drizzle the soy sauce mixture all over, serve, and enjoy!

Extra Air Fried Treats

Perfect Cinnamon Toast

Servings: 6

* 2tsp. Pepper
* 1½ tsp. Vanilla extract
* 1 ½ tsp. Cinnamon
* ½ c. Sweetener of choice
* 1 c. Coconut oil
* 12slices whole wheat bread

Directions:

1.Melt coconut oil and mix with sweetener until dissolved. Mix in remaining minus bread till incorporated.

2.Spread mixture onto bread, covering all area. Place coated pieces of bread in your air fryer.

3.Cook 5 minutes at 400 degrees.

4.Remove and cut diagonally. Enjoy!

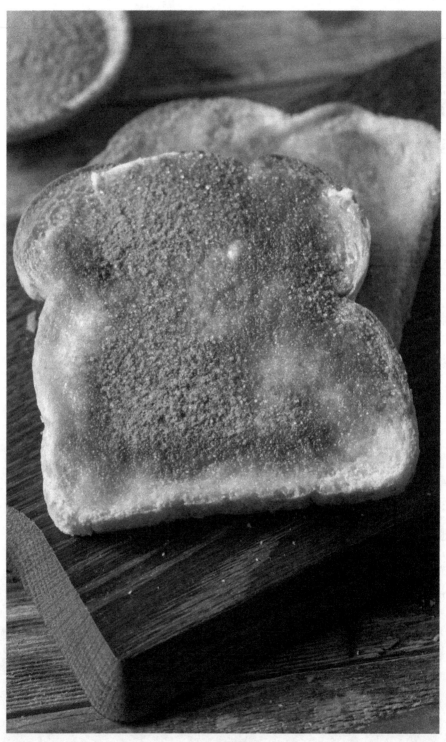

Apple Dumplings

Servings: 4

- 2 tbsp. Melted coconut oil
- 2 puff pastry sheets
- 1 tbsp. Brown Sugar
- 2 tbsp. Raisins
- 2 small apples of choice

Directions:

1. Ensure your air fryer is preheated to 356 degrees.
2. Core and peel apples and mix with raisins and Sugar.
3. Place a bit of apple mixture into puff pastry sheets and brush sides with melted coconut oil.
4. Place into air fryer. Cook 25 minutes, turning halfway through. Will be golden when done.

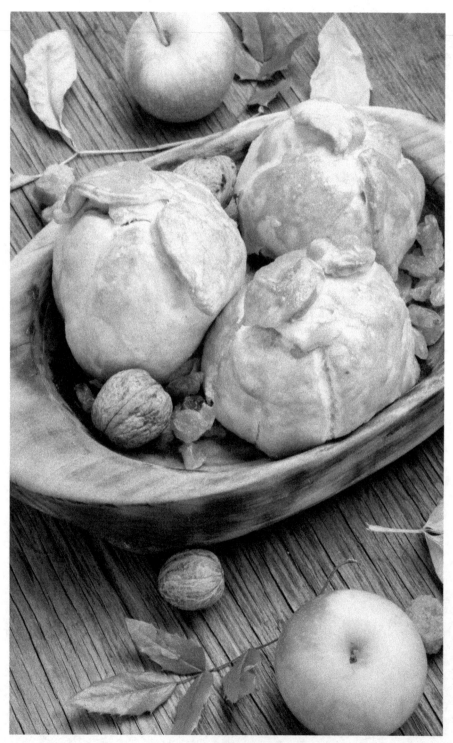

Air Fryer Chocolate Cake

Servings: 8-10

- ½ c. Hot water
- 1 tsp. Vanilla
- ¼ c. Olive oil
- ½ c. Almond milk
- 1 egg
- ½ tsp. Salt
- ¾ tsp. Baking soda
- ¾ tsp. Baking powder
- ½ c. Unsweetened cocoa powder
- 2 c. Almond flour
- c. Brown Sugar

Directions:

1. Preheat your air fryer to 356 degrees.

2. Stir all dry together. Then stir in wet . Add hot water last.

3. The batter will be thin, no worries.

4.Pour cake batter into a pan that fits into the fryer. Cover with foil and poke holes into the foil.

5.Bake 35 minutes.

6.Discard foil and then bake another 10 minutes.

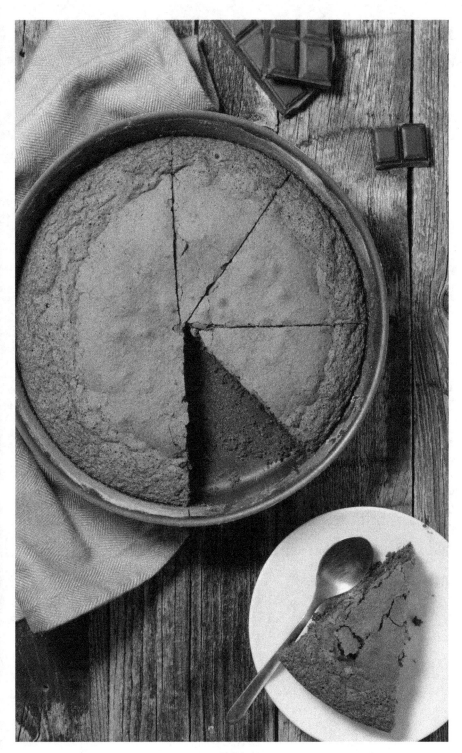

Easy Air Fryer Donuts

Servings: 8

- Pinch of allspice
- 4 tbsp. Dark brown Sugar
- ½ - 1 tsp. Cinnamon
- 1/3 c. Granulated sweetener
- 3 tbsp. Melted coconut oil
- 1 can of biscuits

Directions:

1.Mix allspice, Sugar, sweetener, and cinnamon.

2.Take out biscuits from can and with a circle cookie cutter, cut holes from centers and place into air fryer.

3.Cook 5 minutes at 350 degrees. As batches are cooked, use a brush to coat with melted coconut oil and dip each into Sugar mixture.

4.Serve warm!

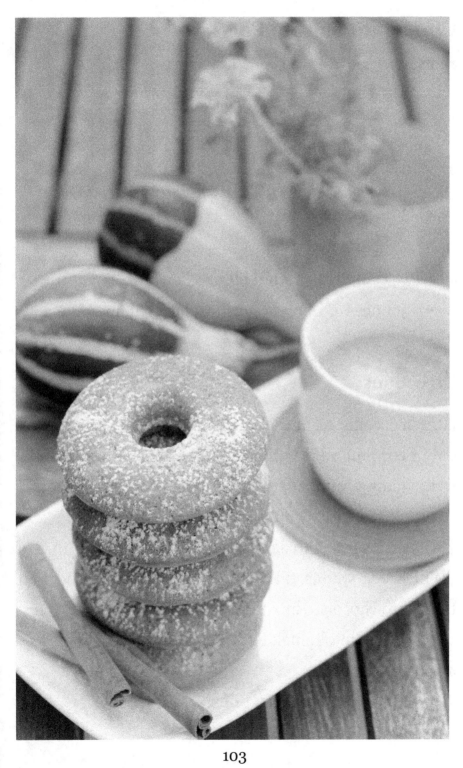

Chocolate Soufflé For Two

Servings: 2

- 2tbsp. Almond flour
- ½ tsp. Vanilla
- 3 tbsp. Sweetener
- 2 separated eggs
- ¼ c. Melted coconut oil
- 3ounces of semi-sweet chocolate, chopped

Directions:

1.Brush coconut oil and sweetener onto ramekins.

2.Melt coconut oil and chocolate together. Beat egg yolks well, adding vanilla and sweetener. Stir in flour and ensure there are no lumps.

3.Preheat fryer to 330 degrees.

4.Whisk egg whites till they reach peak state and fold them into chocolate mixture.

5.Pour batter into ramekins and place into the fryer.

6.Cook 14 minutes.

Serve with powdered Sugar dusted on top.

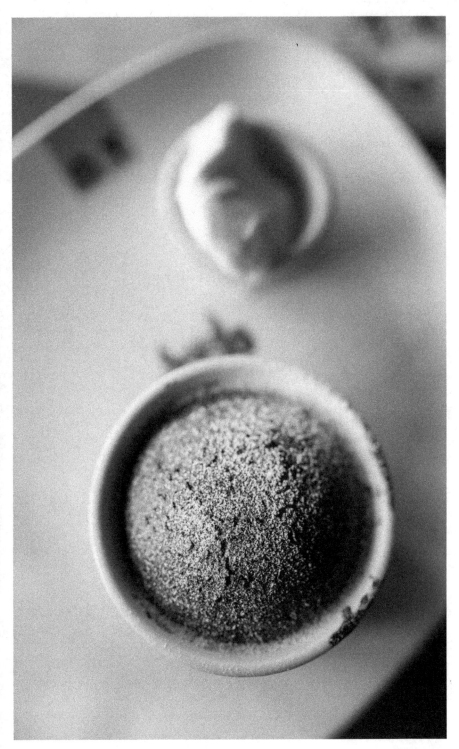

Butter Cake

Serves: 8

- Butter (1 cup)
- Liquid stevia (.25 cup)
- Pure vanilla extract (1 tbsp.)
- Almond flour (3 cups)
- Egg yolks (6) + Whole egg (1 large)
- Salt (.25 tsp.)
- Also Needed: 9-inch springform pan

Directions:

1 Warm the Air Fryer to reach 350° Fahrenheit.

2 Combine the stevia and butter using an electric hand mixer until creamy.

3 Gradually, mix in the yolks and vanilla.

4 Add to the pan, spreading the batter smoothly using a spatula.

5 Put the batter in the refrigerator and wait for about 15 minutes before cooking.

6 Whisk an egg and brush the cake. Air-fry for 35 minutes.

Delicious Blackberry Pie

Serves:8

- Egg (1 large)
- Unsalted butter (2 tbsp.)
- Stevia (1 scoop)
- Baking powder (1 tbsp.)
- Almond flour (1 cup)
- Blackberries (.5 cup)
- Also Needed: Parchment paper

Directions:

1 Warm the Air Fryer to reach 350° Fahrenheit.

2 Whisk the egg, butter, stevia, and baking powder.

3 Reserve 1 teaspoon of the flour and add the rest to the mixture. Knead until smooth – not sticky.

4 Cover the fryer basket using a layer of baking paper and add the dough. Flatten into a pie crust and add the berries. Sprinkle with the rest of the almond flour on top.

5 Air-fry until it's golden or about 20 minutes. Chill before slicing to serve.

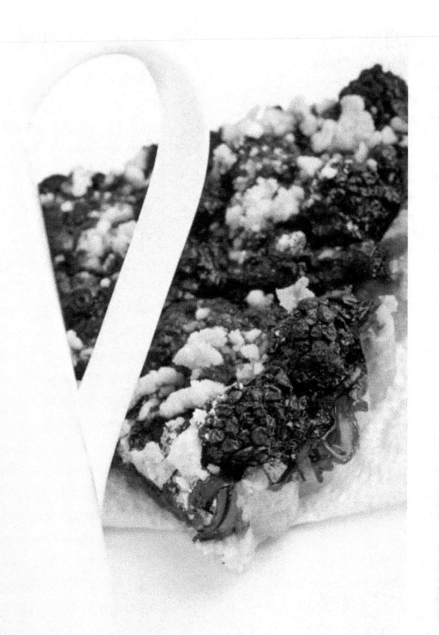